THE ACID REFLUX COOKBOOK

Delicious and Nutritious Dishes to Relieve Discomfort

T. John

COPYRIGHT PAGE

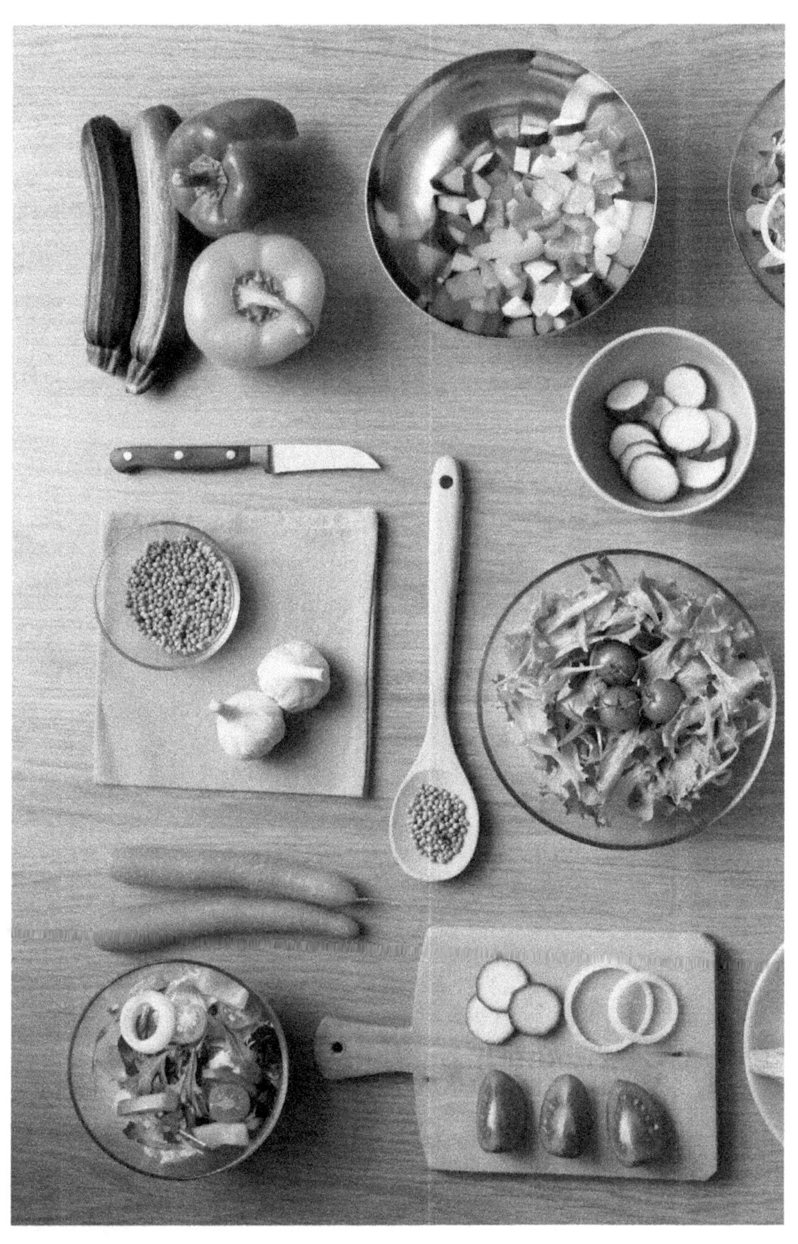

TABLE OF CONTENTS

INTRODUCTION

Welcome to "The Acid Reflux Cookbook," your ultimate guide to managing acid reflux through delicious and wholesome recipes. In this introductory chapter, we will lay the foundation for your journey towards better digestive health. We'll explore the impact of acid reflux on your well-being and introduce you to the benefits of adopting an acid reflux diet. Let's dive in!

Understanding Acid Reflux and its Impact on Your Health

Acid reflux, also known as gastroesophageal reflux disease (GERD), is a condition characterized by the backflow of stomach acid into the esophagus. This can lead to a range of uncomfortable symptoms, including heartburn, regurgitation, and chest pain. To better understand the impact of acid reflux on your health, let's delve into the underlying causes and potential complications.

The Causes of Acid Reflux

Acid reflux is primarily caused by a malfunctioning lower esophageal sphincter (LES), a muscular valve that separates the esophagus from the stomach. When the LES weakens or relaxes inappropriately, stomach acid can flow back into the esophagus, leading to acid reflux symptoms. Factors such as obesity, certain foods, smoking, and certain medications can contribute to the development of acid reflux.

The Symptoms of Acid Reflux

Recognizing the symptoms of acid reflux is crucial for proper diagnosis and treatment. Typical signs of acid reflux include heartburn, a burning sensation in the chest, regurgitation of acidic fluid or food, difficulty swallowing, and a persistent cough. It's important to consult with a healthcare professional to accurately diagnose acid reflux and differentiate it from other conditions with similar symptoms.

Potential Complications of Acid Reflux

While acid reflux symptoms can be distressing, untreated or poorly managed acid reflux can lead to more severe complications. Chronic acid reflux can cause inflammation and damage to the lining of the esophagus, increasing the risk of developing esophageal ulcers, strictures, and even Barrett's esophagus, a condition that may progress to esophageal cancer. Early intervention and lifestyle modifications are essential for preventing these complications.

How This Cookbook Can Help You Manage Acid Reflux

"The Acid Reflux Cookbook" is designed to empower you with the knowledge and recipes needed to effectively manage acid reflux and promote a healthy digestive system. Let's explore how this cookbook can become your trusted companion in your acid reflux journey.

This cookbook adopts a holistic approach to acid reflux management, focusing not only on dietary modifications but also on lifestyle changes and overall well-being. By addressing the root causes and triggers of acid reflux, we aim to provide you with a comprehensive toolkit for long-term relief.

Diet plays a pivotal role in managing acid reflux. Certain foods can exacerbate symptoms, while others can help alleviate discomfort and promote healing. Throughout this cookbook, we will explore the foods to avoid and include in your acid reflux diet, as well as tips for mindful eating and portion control.

Chapter 1: The Acid Reflux Diet Basics

Foods to Avoid to Minimize Acid Reflux Symptoms

Certain foods and beverages are known to trigger or exacerbate acid reflux symptoms. Understanding which foods to avoid can significantly alleviate discomfort and promote better digestive health. Here are some key culprits that should be limited or eliminated from your diet:

1. Citrus Fruits: Oranges, lemons, grapefruits, and their juices are highly acidic and can aggravate acid reflux symptoms. Opt for less acidic alternatives like apples and bananas.

2. Tomatoes and Tomato-based Products: Tomatoes are naturally acidic, and foods like tomato sauce, ketchup, and salsa can trigger acid reflux. Consider using alternative sauces or limiting your tomato consumption.

3. Spicy Foods: Spices such as chili powder, black pepper, and hot peppers can irritate the esophagus and worsen acid reflux symptoms. Choose milder seasonings or spices that don't cause discomfort.

4. Fatty and Fried Foods: High-fat foods, like fried foods and fatty cuts of meat, take longer to digest and can increase the risk of acid reflux. Opt for leaner protein sources and cooking methods like grilling or baking.

5. Carbonated Beverages: Carbonated drinks, including soda and sparkling water, can cause bloating and increase pressure on the stomach, leading to acid reflux. Choose non-carbonated alternatives like herbal tea or water.

Foods to Include for a Healthy Digestive System

While certain foods can trigger acid reflux, others can help soothe the digestive system and reduce symptoms. By incorporating these foods into your diet, you can support better digestion and minimize acid reflux discomfort:

1. Non-Citrus Fruits: Apples, bananas, melons, and pears are excellent choices that provide essential nutrients while being gentle on the stomach.

2. Vegetables: Incorporate a variety of vegetables into your meals, including leafy greens like spinach and kale, broccoli, cauliflower, carrots, and cucumbers.

3. Lean Protein: Opt for lean protein sources such as chicken breast, turkey, fish, and tofu. These provide essential nutrients without the added fat that can trigger acid reflux.

4. Whole Grains: Choose whole grain options like brown rice, quinoa, oatmeal, and whole wheat bread, which are rich in fiber and promote healthy digestion.

5. Healthy Fats: Include sources of healthy fats in your diet, such as avocados, olive oil, nuts, and seeds. These fats support overall health and do not typically trigger acid reflux.

Lifestyle Modifications to Support Acid Reflux Management

In addition to dietary changes, certain lifestyle modifications can significantly contribute to managing acid reflux symptoms. Implementing the following practices can promote better digestion and reduce the likelihood of acid reflux:

1. Portion Control: Eating smaller, more frequent meals rather than large portions can help prevent excessive pressure on the stomach and reduce the risk of acid reflux.

2. Slow Eating and Mindful Eating: Chew your food thoroughly and savor each bite. Eating slowly and mindfully allows your body to properly digest the food and helps prevent overeating.

3. Maintain a Healthy Weight: Excess weight can increase pressure on the abdomen and contribute to acid reflux. Engage in regular physical activity and adopt a well-balanced diet to maintain a healthy weight.

4. Avoid Triggering Activities: Certain activities, such as lying down or bending over after meals, can worsen acid reflux symptoms. Maintain an upright position for at least two to three hours after eating.

5. Elevate the Head of Your Bed: Elevating the head of your bed by a few inches can help prevent stomach acid from flowing back into the esophagus while you sleep.

Chapter 2: 30 Day Meal Plan

Here's a 30-day meal plan incorporating the provided recipes:

Day 1:

Breakfast: Scrambled Tofu Breakfast Bowl

Lunch: Grilled Chicken and Vegetable Salad

Dinner: Baked Lemon Herb Chicken

Snack: Roasted Red Pepper Hummus with Crudité

Dessert: Berry Chia Pudding

Smoothie: Green Detox Smoothie

Day 2:

Breakfast: Oatmeal with Fresh Berries and Almonds

Lunch: Turkey and Avocado Wrap

Dinner: Beef Stir-Fry with Broccoli and Bell Peppers

Snack: Guacamole with Baked Tortilla Chips

Dessert: Baked Apples with Cinnamon and Almonds

Smoothie: Banana Berry Smoothie

Day 3:

Breakfast: Spinach and Mushroom Egg Muffins

Lunch: Quinoa and Roasted Vegetable Bowl

Dinner: Grilled Salmon with Dill Sauce

Snack: Greek Yogurt and Fruit Dip

Dessert: Coconut Yogurt Parfait with Mixed Berries

Smoothie: Tropical Turmeric Smoothie

Day 4:

Breakfast: Blueberry Banana Pancakes

Lunch: Salmon and Asparagus Foil Pack

Dinner: Shrimp and Vegetable Stir-Fry

Snack: Cucumber and Tomato Bruschetta

Dessert: Chocolate Avocado Mousse

Smoothie: Spinach and Pineapple Smoothie

Day 5:

Breakfast: Avocado Toast with Smoked Salmon

Lunch: Mediterranean Chickpea Salad

Dinner: Roasted Turkey Breast with Sweet Potatoes

Snack: Baked Sweet Potato Fries

Dessert: Almond Flour Banana Bread

Smoothie: Mango Ginger Smoothie

Day 6:

Breakfast: Quinoa Breakfast Porridge

Lunch: Caprese Skewers with Balsamic Glaze

Dinner: Quinoa Stuffed Bell Peppers

Snack: Oven-Baked Zucchini Chips

Dessert: Mango Sorbet

Smoothie: Blueberry Avocado Smoothie

Day 7:

Breakfast: Vegetable and Egg Wrap

Lunch: Zucchini Noodles with Pesto and Cherry Tomatoes

Dinner: Eggplant Parmesan

Snack: Stuffed Mushrooms with Spinach and Feta

Dessert: Grilled Pineapple with Honey and Mint

Smoothie: Raspberry Beet Smoothie

Day 8:

Breakfast: Greek Yogurt Parfait with Granola

Lunch: Tuna Salad Lettuce Wraps

Dinner: Vegetable Curry with Brown Rice

Snack: Quinoa and Black Bean Salad Cups

Dessert: Roasted Peaches with Greek Yogurt

Smoothie: Kiwi Kale Smoothie

Day 9:

Breakfast: Almond Butter and Banana Smoothie Bowl

Lunch: Lentil Soup with Vegetables

Dinner: Mexican Cauliflower Rice Bowl

Snack: Smoked Salmon Roll-Ups

Dessert: Strawberry Almond Crumble

Smoothie: Papaya Passion Smoothie

Day 10:

Breakfast: Veggie Omelette with Whole Grain Toast

Lunch: Greek Salad with Grilled Shrimp

Dinner: Baked Cod with Lemon and Herbs

Snack: Spicy Edamame

Dessert: Blueberry Coconut Ice Cream

Smoothie: Almond Butter and Chocolate Smoothie

Day 11:

Breakfast: Scrambled Tofu Breakfast Bowl

Lunch: Grilled Chicken and Vegetable Salad

Dinner: Baked Lemon Herb Chicken

Snack: Roasted Red Pepper Hummus with Crudité

Dessert: Berry Chia Pudding

Smoothie: Green Detox Smoothie

Day 12:

Breakfast: Oatmeal with Fresh Berries and Almonds

Lunch: Turkey and Avocado Wrap

Dinner: Beef Stir-Fry with Broccoli and Bell Peppers

Snack: Guacamole with Baked Tortilla Chips

Dessert: Baked Apples with Cinnamon and Almonds

Smoothie: Banana Berry Smoothie

Day 13:

Breakfast: Spinach and Mushroom Egg Muffins

Lunch: Quinoa and Roasted Vegetable Bowl

Dinner: Grilled Salmon with Dill Sauce

Snack: Greek Yogurt and Fruit Dip

Dessert: Coconut Yogurt Parfait with Mixed Berries

Smoothie: Tropical Turmeric Smoothie

Day 14:

Breakfast: Blueberry Banana Pancakes

Lunch: Salmon and Asparagus Foil Pack

Dinner: Shrimp and Vegetable Stir-Fry

Snack: Cucumber and Tomato Bruschetta

Dessert: Chocolate Avocado Mousse

Smoothie: Spinach and Pineapple Smoothie

Day 15:

Breakfast: Avocado Toast with Smoked Salmon

Lunch: Mediterranean Chickpea Salad

Dinner: Roasted Turkey Breast with Sweet Potatoes

Snack: Baked Sweet Potato Fries

Dessert: Almond Flour Banana Bread

Smoothie: Mango Ginger Smoothie

Day 16:

Breakfast: Quinoa Breakfast Porridge

Lunch: Caprese Skewers with Balsamic Glaze

Dinner: Quinoa Stuffed Bell Peppers

Snack: Oven-Baked Zucchini Chips

Dessert: Mango Sorbet

Smoothie: Blueberry Avocado Smoothie

Day 17:

Breakfast: Vegetable and Egg Wrap

Lunch: Zucchini Noodles with Pesto and Cherry Tomatoes

Dinner: Eggplant Parmesan

Snack: Stuffed Mushrooms with Spinach and Feta

Dessert: Grilled Pineapple with Honey and Mint

Smoothie: Raspberry Beet Smoothie

Day 18:

Breakfast: Greek Yogurt Parfait with Granola

Lunch: Tuna Salad Lettuce Wraps

Dinner: Vegetable Curry with Brown Rice

Snack: Quinoa and Black Bean Salad Cups

Dessert: Roasted Peaches with Greek Yogurt

Smoothie: Kiwi Kale Smoothie

Day 19:

Breakfast: Almond Butter and Banana Smoothie Bowl

Lunch: Lentil Soup with Vegetables

Dinner: Mexican Cauliflower Rice Bowl

Snack: Smoked Salmon Roll-Ups

Dessert: Strawberry Almond Crumble

Smoothie: Papaya Passion Smoothie

Day 20:

Breakfast: Veggie Omelette with Whole Grain Toast

Lunch: Greek Salad with Grilled Shrimp

Dinner: Baked Cod with Lemon and Herbs

Snack: Spicy Edamame

Dessert: Blueberry Coconut Ice Cream

Smoothie: Almond Butter and Chocolate Smoothie

Day 21:

Breakfast: Scrambled Tofu Breakfast Bowl

Lunch: Grilled Chicken and Vegetable Salad

Dinner: Baked Lemon Herb Chicken

Snack: Roasted Red Pepper Hummus with Crudité

Dessert: Berry Chia Pudding

Smoothie: Green Detox Smoothie

Day 22:

Breakfast: Oatmeal with Fresh Berries and Almonds

Lunch: Turkey and Avocado Wrap

Dinner: Beef Stir-Fry with Broccoli and Bell Peppers

Snack: Guacamole with Baked Tortilla Chips

Dessert: Baked Apples with Cinnamon and Almonds

Smoothie: Banana Berry Smoothie

Day 23:

Breakfast: Spinach and Mushroom Egg Muffins

Lunch: Quinoa and Roasted Vegetable Bowl

Dinner: Grilled Salmon with Dill Sauce

Snack: Greek Yogurt and Fruit Dip

Dessert: Coconut Yogurt Parfait with Mixed Berries

Smoothie: Tropical Turmeric Smoothie

Day 24:

Breakfast: Blueberry Banana Pancakes

Lunch: Salmon and Asparagus Foil Pack

Dinner: Shrimp and Vegetable Stir-Fry

Snack: Cucumber and Tomato Bruschetta

Dessert: Chocolate Avocado Mousse

Smoothie: Spinach and Pineapple Smoothie

Day 25:

Breakfast: Avocado Toast with Smoked Salmon

Lunch: Mediterranean Chickpea Salad

Dinner: Roasted Turkey Breast with Sweet Potatoes

Snack: Baked Sweet Potato Fries

Dessert: Almond Flour Banana Bread

Smoothie: Mango Ginger Smoothie

Day 26:

Breakfast: Quinoa Breakfast Porridge

Lunch: Caprese Skewers with Balsamic Glaze

Dinner: Quinoa Stuffed Bell Peppers

Snack: Oven-Baked Zucchini Chips

Dessert: Mango Sorbet

Smoothie: Blueberry Avocado Smoothie

Day 27:

Breakfast: Vegetable and Egg Wrap

Lunch: Zucchini Noodles with Pesto and Cherry Tomatoes

Dinner: Eggplant Parmesan

Snack: Stuffed Mushrooms with Spinach and Feta

Dessert: Grilled Pineapple with Honey and Mint

Smoothie: Raspberry Beet Smoothie

Day 28:

Breakfast: Greek Yogurt Parfait with Granola

Lunch: Tuna Salad Lettuce Wraps

Dinner: Vegetable Curry with Brown Rice

Snack: Quinoa and Black Bean Salad Cups

Dessert: Roasted Peaches with Greek Yogurt

Smoothie: Kiwi Kale Smoothie

Day 29:

Breakfast: Almond Butter and Banana Smoothie Bowl

Lunch: Lentil Soup with Vegetables

Dinner: Mexican Cauliflower Rice Bowl

Snack: Smoked Salmon Roll-Ups

Dessert: Strawberry Almond Crumble

Smoothie: Papaya Passion Smoothie

Day 30:

Breakfast: Veggie Omelette with Whole Grain Toast

Lunch: Greek Salad with Grilled Shrimp

Dinner: Baked Cod with Lemon and Herbs

Snack: Spicy Edamame

Dessert: Blueberry Coconut Ice Cream

Smoothie: Almond Butter and Chocolate Smoothie

Chapter 3: Breakfast Recipes

In this chapter, we will explore a variety of delicious and nutritious breakfast recipes that are perfect for starting your day on a healthy note. These recipes are designed to be both satisfying and gentle on the digestive system, making them ideal for individuals managing acid reflux. Let's dive into these mouthwatering breakfast options:

Scrambled Tofu Breakfast Bowl

Ingredients:

- 1 tablespoon olive oil
- 1/2 cup diced bell peppers
- 1/4 cup diced onions
- 1 cup crumbled tofu
- 1/2 teaspoon turmeric
- 1/4 teaspoon garlic powder
- Salt and pepper to taste
- Fresh parsley, chopped (for garnish)

Instructions:

1. Heat olive oil in a skillet over medium heat.

2. Add bell peppers and onions, and sauté until softened.

3. Crumble the tofu into the skillet and stir well.

4. Sprinkle turmeric, garlic powder, salt, and pepper over the tofu mixture.

5. Cook for 5-7 minutes, stirring occasionally, until the tofu is heated through and lightly golden.

6. Transfer the scrambled tofu to a bowl and garnish with fresh parsley.

7. Serve warm and enjoy this protein-packed breakfast!

Oatmeal with Fresh Berries and Almonds

Ingredients:

- 1/2 cup rolled oats
- 1 cup water or milk (dairy or plant-based)
- 1/2 cup mixed fresh berries (such as strawberries, blueberries, and raspberries)
- 2 tablespoons sliced almonds
- 1 tablespoon honey or maple syrup (optional)

Instructions:

1. In a saucepan, bring water or milk to a boil.
2. Add rolled oats and reduce heat to low. Cook for 5 minutes, stirring occasionally.
3. Once the oats have thickened, remove the saucepan from heat.
4. Transfer the cooked oats to a bowl and top with fresh berries and sliced almonds.
5. Drizzle honey or maple syrup over the oatmeal if desired for added sweetness.
6. Stir gently to combine the ingredients.
7. Enjoy a warm and comforting bowl of oatmeal to kick-start your day!

Spinach and Mushroom Egg Muffins

Ingredients:

- 6 large eggs
- 1 cup spinach, chopped
- 1/2 cup sliced mushrooms
- 1/4 cup diced onions
- Salt and pepper to taste
- Cooking spray or olive oil for greasing

Instructions:

1. Preheat the oven to 350°F (175°C). Grease a muffin tin with cooking spray or olive oil.
2. In a bowl, whisk the eggs until well beaten.
3. Add chopped spinach, sliced mushrooms, diced onions, salt, and pepper to the bowl. Mix well.
4. Pour the egg mixture evenly into the prepared muffin tin, filling each cup about 3/4 full.
5. Bake for 15-20 minutes, or until the egg muffins are set and lightly golden on top.
6. Remove from the oven and let cool for a few minutes before removing from the muffin tin.
7. Serve warm and savor these portable and nutritious egg muffins!

Blueberry Banana Pancakes

Ingredients:

- 1 cup whole wheat flour
- 1 tablespoon baking powder
- 1/4 teaspoon salt
- 1 ripe banana, mashed
- 1 cup almond milk (or any milk of your choice)

- 1 tablespoon honey or maple syrup
- 1/2 cup fresh blueberries
- Cooking spray or butter for greasing

Instructions:

1. In a mixing bowl, combine whole wheat flour, baking powder, and salt.
2. In a separate bowl, whisk together mashed banana, almond milk, and honey or maple syrup.
3. Pour the wet ingredients into the dry ingredients and stir until just combined. Be careful not to overmix.
4. Gently fold in the fresh blueberries.
5. Heat a non-stick skillet or griddle over medium heat and lightly grease with cooking spray or butter.
6. Spoon about 1/4 cup of batter onto the skillet for each pancake.
7. Cook until bubbles form on the surface, then flip and cook the other side until golden brown.
8. Repeat with the remaining batter.
9. Serve these fluffy blueberry banana pancakes with a drizzle of honey or maple syrup on top.

Avocado Toast with Smoked Salmon

Ingredients:

- 2 slices whole grain bread, toasted
- 1 ripe avocado
- Juice of 1/2 lemon
- Salt and pepper to taste
- 2 ounces smoked salmon
- Fresh dill, chopped (for garnish)

Instructions:

1. In a bowl, mash the ripe avocado with lemon juice, salt, and pepper until smooth.
2. Spread the avocado mixture evenly onto the toasted bread slices.
3. Top each slice with smoked salmon.
4. Garnish with fresh dill.
5. Serve this satisfying avocado toast with smoked salmon for a nutritious and flavorful breakfast.

Quinoa Breakfast Porridge

Ingredients:

- 1/2 cup quinoa, rinsed

- 1 cup water or milk (dairy or plant-based)
- 1/4 teaspoon ground cinnamon
- 1 tablespoon honey or maple syrup
- 1/4 cup chopped nuts (such as almonds, walnuts, or pecans)
- Fresh berries for topping

Instructions:

1. In a saucepan, combine quinoa, water or milk, and ground cinnamon.
2. Bring the mixture to a boil, then reduce heat to low and cover.
3. Simmer for 15-20 minutes, or until the quinoa is cooked and has absorbed the liquid.
4. Remove from heat and let stand for a few minutes.
5. Stir in honey or maple syrup and chopped nuts.
6. Transfer the quinoa porridge to serving bowls and top with fresh berries.
7. Enjoy this wholesome and protein-packed breakfast porridge!

Vegetable and Egg Wrap

Ingredients:

- 2 large eggs
- 1/4 cup diced bell peppers
- 1/4 cup diced onions
- 1/4 cup sliced mushrooms
- 1/4 cup spinach leaves
- Salt and pepper to taste
- 2 whole grain tortillas

Instructions:

1. In a bowl, whisk the eggs until well beaten.
2. Heat a non-stick skillet over medium heat and lightly grease with cooking spray or olive oil.
3. Add bell peppers, onions, and mushrooms to the skillet. Sauté until softened.
4. Add spinach leaves and cook until wilted.
5. Pour the beaten eggs into the skillet and scramble them with the vegetables. Season with salt and pepper.
6. Warm the tortillas in a separate skillet or microwave.

7. Spoon the scrambled egg and vegetable mixture onto each tortilla, then roll it up into a wrap.

8. Cut the wraps in half and serve as a satisfying and nutritious breakfast option.

Greek Yogurt Parfait with Granola

Ingredients:

- 1 cup Greek yogurt
- 1/2 cup mixed fresh berries (such as blueberries, raspberries, and strawberries)
- 1/4 cup granola
- 1 tablespoon honey or maple syrup (optional)

Instructions:

1. In a glass or bowl, layer Greek yogurt, fresh berries, and granola.

2. Repeat the layers until all ingredients are used.

3. Drizzle honey or maple syrup over the top if desired for added sweetness.

4. Enjoy this creamy and crunchy Greek yogurt parfait as a refreshing breakfast treat.

Almond Butter and Banana Smoothie Bowl

Ingredients:

- 2 ripe bananas, frozen and sliced
- 1/4 cup almond butter
- 1/2 cup almond milk (or any milk of your choice)
- 1 tablespoon honey or maple syrup
- Toppings: sliced banana, chopped nuts, shredded coconut, chia seeds (optional)

Instructions:

1. In a blender, combine frozen banana slices, almond butter, almond milk, and honey or maple syrup.
2. Blend until smooth and creamy.
3. Pour the smoothie into a bowl.
4. Top with sliced banana, chopped nuts, shredded coconut, and chia seeds if desired.
5. Enjoy this luscious almond butter and banana smoothie bowl as a nutritious and energizing breakfast.

Veggie Omelette with Whole Grain Toast

Ingredients:

- 3 large eggs
- 2 tablespoons diced bell peppers
- 2 tablespoons diced onions
- 2 tablespoons sliced mushrooms
- 2 tablespoons chopped spinach leaves
- Salt and pepper to taste
- Cooking spray or olive oil for greasing
- 2 slices whole grain toast

Instructions:

1. In a bowl, whisk the eggs until well beaten.
2. Heat a non-stick skillet over medium heat and lightly grease with cooking spray or olive oil.
3. Add bell peppers, onions, and mushrooms to the skillet. Sauté until softened.
4. Add chopped spinach leaves and cook until wilted.
5. Pour the beaten eggs into the skillet, covering the vegetables. Season with salt and pepper.
6. Cook until the omelette is set, then fold it in half.

7. Remove the omelette from the skillet and serve with whole grain toast on the side.

8. Enjoy this hearty and veggie-packed omelette as a satisfying breakfast option.

Chapter 4: Lunch Recipes

In this chapter, we will explore a variety of delicious and nutritious lunch recipes that are specifically designed to be gentle on your digestive system while still satisfying your taste buds. These recipes are carefully crafted to help alleviate the symptoms of acid reflux and promote a healthy gut. Let's dive in and discover these delightful lunch options!

Grilled Chicken and Vegetable Salad

Ingredients:

- 2 boneless, skinless chicken breasts
- 1 tablespoon olive oil
- Salt and pepper to taste
- 4 cups mixed salad greens
- 1 cup cherry tomatoes, halved
- 1 cucumber, sliced
- 1 bell pepper, sliced
- 1/4 cup red onion, thinly sliced
- 1/4 cup feta cheese, crumbled
- 2 tablespoons lemon juice

- 1 tablespoon balsamic vinegar

Instructions:

1. Preheat the grill to medium-high heat.
2. Brush the chicken breasts with olive oil and season with salt and pepper.
3. Grill the chicken for about 6-8 minutes per side, or until cooked through. Remove from heat and let it rest for a few minutes before slicing.
4. In a large bowl, combine the salad greens, cherry tomatoes, cucumber, bell pepper, red onion, and feta cheese.
5. In a small bowl, whisk together the lemon juice and balsamic vinegar. Drizzle the dressing over the salad and toss to combine.
6. Slice the grilled chicken and arrange it on top of the salad. Serve and enjoy!

Turkey and Avocado Wrap

Ingredients:

- 4 whole wheat tortillas
- 8 slices turkey breast

- 1 avocado, sliced
- 1/2 cup spinach leaves
- 1/4 cup sliced red onion
- 2 tablespoons Greek yogurt
- 1 tablespoon Dijon mustard
- Salt and pepper to taste

Instructions:

1. Lay out the tortillas and divide the turkey breast, avocado slices, spinach leaves, and red onion equally among them.

2. In a small bowl, mix together the Greek yogurt, Dijon mustard, salt, and pepper. Spread the mixture evenly on each tortilla.

3. Roll up the tortillas tightly, enclosing the filling. Cut each wrap in half and secure with toothpicks if needed.

4. Serve the turkey and avocado wraps immediately or refrigerate until ready to eat. Enjoy as a quick and satisfying lunch!

Quinoa and Roasted Vegetable Bowl

Ingredients:

- 1 cup cooked quinoa
- 1 cup roasted vegetables (such as zucchini, bell peppers, and carrots)
- 1/4 cup crumbled goat cheese
- 2 tablespoons chopped fresh basil
- 1 tablespoon lemon juice
- 1 tablespoon extra virgin olive oil
- Salt and pepper to taste

Instructions:

1. In a bowl, combine the cooked quinoa and roasted vegetables.
2. Add the crumbled goat cheese and chopped basil to the bowl.
3. In a small container, whisk together the lemon juice, olive oil, salt, and pepper. Pour the dressing over the quinoa and vegetable mixture.
4. Toss gently to combine all the ingredients.

5. Serve the quinoa and roasted vegetable bowl at room temperature or chilled. It makes a hearty and nutritious lunch option.

Salmon and Asparagus Foil Pack

Ingredients:

- 2 salmon fillets
- 1 bunch asparagus, trimmed
- 1 lemon, sliced
- 2 tablespoons melted butter
- 2 cloves garlic, minced
- 1 tablespoon chopped fresh dill
- Salt and pepper to taste

Instructions:

1. Preheat the oven to 400°F (200°C).
2. Place each salmon fillet on a separate piece of aluminum foil.
3. Arrange the trimmed asparagus around the salmon.
4. Top the salmon and asparagus with lemon slices.

5. In a small bowl, mix together the melted butter, minced garlic, chopped dill, salt, and pepper. Drizzle the mixture over the salmon and asparagus.

6. Fold the foil to create a sealed packet, ensuring that the contents are tightly enclosed.

7. Place the foil packets on a baking sheet and bake in the preheated oven for about 15-20 minutes, or until the salmon is cooked through and the asparagus is tender.

8. Carefully open the foil packets and transfer the salmon and asparagus to a plate. Serve and enjoy the flavorful combination!

Mediterranean Chickpea Salad

Ingredients:

- 2 cups canned chickpeas, rinsed and drained
- 1 cup cherry tomatoes, halved
- 1 cucumber, diced
- 1/4 cup red onion, finely chopped
- 1/4 cup Kalamata olives, pitted and halved
- 1/4 cup crumbled feta cheese
- 2 tablespoons chopped fresh parsley

- 2 tablespoons lemon juice
- 1 tablespoon extra virgin olive oil
- 1 clove garlic, minced
- Salt and pepper to taste

Instructions:

1. In a large bowl, combine the chickpeas, cherry tomatoes, cucumber, red onion, Kalamata olives, feta cheese, and chopped parsley.
2. In a small container, whisk together the lemon juice, olive oil, minced garlic, salt, and pepper. Pour the dressing over the salad ingredients.
3. Toss gently to coat all the ingredients with the dressing.
4. Let the Mediterranean chickpea salad sit for about 10 minutes to allow the flavors to meld together.
5. Serve the salad as a refreshing and protein-packed lunch option.

Caprese Skewers with Balsamic Glaze

Ingredients:

- 12 cherry tomatoes
- 12 small mozzarella balls
- 12 fresh basil leaves
- Balsamic glaze for drizzling
- Salt and pepper to taste

Instructions:

1. Thread a cherry tomato, mozzarella ball, and fresh basil leaf onto a skewer. Repeat with the remaining ingredients to assemble all the skewers.
2. Arrange the caprese skewers on a serving platter.
3. Drizzle the skewers with balsamic glaze and sprinkle with salt and pepper.
4. Serve the caprese skewers as a delightful and visually appealing lunch option. The combination of flavors is sure to please your taste buds.

Zucchini Noodles with Pesto and Cherry Tomatoes

Ingredients:

- 2 medium zucchinis
- 1 cup cherry tomatoes, halved

- 1/4 cup pine nuts, toasted
- 2 tablespoons grated Parmesan cheese
- 1 cup fresh basil leaves
- 1 clove garlic
- 1/4 cup extra virgin olive oil
- Salt and pepper to taste

Instructions:

1. Using a spiralizer or a julienne peeler, turn the zucchinis into noodles.
2. In a food processor, combine the toasted pine nuts, grated Parmesan cheese, basil leaves, garlic, olive oil, salt, and pepper. Process until smooth to create the pesto sauce.
3. In a large skillet, heat a tablespoon of olive oil over medium heat. Add the zucchini noodles and sauté for 2-3 minutes until tender.
4. Add the cherry tomatoes to the skillet and cook for an additional minute.
5. Remove the skillet from heat and toss the zucchini noodles and cherry tomatoes with the pesto sauce.

6. Serve the zucchini noodles with pesto and cherry tomatoes as a light and flavorful lunch option.

Tuna Salad Lettuce Wraps

Ingredients:

- 2 cans tuna, drained
- 1/4 cup Greek yogurt
- 2 tablespoons mayonnaise
- 1 celery stalk, finely chopped
- 2 tablespoons chopped red onion
- 1 tablespoon chopped fresh dill
- 1 tablespoon lemon juice
- Salt and pepper to taste
- Lettuce leaves for wrapping

Instructions:

1. In a bowl, combine the drained tuna, Greek yogurt, mayonnaise, chopped celery, chopped red onion, chopped dill, lemon juice, salt, and pepper. Mix well to incorporate all the ingredients.

2. Place a spoonful of the tuna salad onto a lettuce leaf.

3. Roll up the lettuce leaf, enclosing the filling, and secure with toothpicks if needed.

4. Repeat with the remaining lettuce leaves and tuna salad mixture.

5. Serve the tuna salad lettuce wraps as a light and protein-rich lunch option. Enjoy the satisfying crunch of lettuce combined with the flavorful tuna salad.

Lentil Soup with Vegetables

Ingredients:

- 1 cup dried lentils
- 1 onion, diced
- 2 carrots, diced
- 2 celery stalks, diced
- 2 cloves garlic, minced
- 4 cups vegetable broth
- 1 teaspoon cumin
- 1 teaspoon paprika
- 1/2 teaspoon turmeric
- Salt and pepper to taste
- Fresh parsley for garnish

Instructions:

1. Rinse the lentils under cold water and drain.

2. In a large pot, sauté the diced onion, carrots, celery, and minced garlic until they soften and become fragrant.

3. Add the rinsed lentils, vegetable broth, cumin, paprika, turmeric, salt, and pepper to the pot. Stir to combine all the ingredients.

4. Bring the soup to a boil, then reduce the heat and let it simmer for about 30-40 minutes, or until the lentils are tender.

5. Adjust the seasonings to taste, adding more salt and pepper if desired.

6. Ladle the lentil soup into bowls, garnish with fresh parsley, and serve it as a nourishing and comforting lunch option.

Greek Salad with Grilled Shrimp

Ingredients:

- 1 pound shrimp, peeled and deveined
- 2 tablespoons olive oil
- 1 teaspoon dried oregano

- 1 teaspoon garlic powder
- Salt and pepper to taste
- 4 cups mixed salad greens
- 1 cucumber, sliced
- 1 cup cherry tomatoes, halved
- 1/2 cup Kalamata olives, pitted
- 1/4 cup sliced red onion
- 1/4 cup crumbled feta cheese
- 2 tablespoons lemon juice
- 1 tablespoon extra virgin olive oil

Instructions:

1. In a bowl, toss the shrimp with olive oil, dried oregano, garlic powder, salt, and pepper.
2. Preheat the grill to medium-high heat. Grill the shrimp for about 2-3 minutes per side, or until they turn pink and opaque. Remove from heat.
3. In a large salad bowl, combine the mixed salad greens, cucumber slices, cherry tomatoes, Kalamata olives, sliced red onion, and crumbled feta cheese.

4. In a small container, whisk together the lemon juice and extra virgin olive oil. Drizzle the dressing over the salad and toss gently to coat all the ingredients.

5. Add the grilled shrimp to the salad and toss lightly.

6. Serve the Greek salad with grilled shrimp as a satisfying and protein-packed lunch option. The combination of fresh ingredients and flavorful shrimp will leave you feeling satisfied and nourished.

Chapter 5: Dinner Recipes

In this chapter, we will explore a variety of delicious and nutritious dinner recipes that are not only satisfying but also suitable for individuals with acid reflux. These recipes focus on using ingredients that are gentle on the digestive system while still offering robust flavors and wholesome ingredients. Let's dive into these ten mouthwatering dinner options.

Baked Lemon Herb Chicken

Ingredients:

- 4 boneless, skinless chicken breasts
- 2 tablespoons olive oil
- 2 tablespoons fresh lemon juice
- 2 cloves garlic, minced
- 1 teaspoon dried thyme
- 1 teaspoon dried rosemary
- Salt and pepper to taste

Instructions:

1. Preheat the oven to 375°F (190°C).

2. In a small bowl, combine the olive oil, lemon juice, minced garlic, dried thyme, dried rosemary, salt, and pepper.

3. Place the chicken breasts in a baking dish and pour the lemon herb mixture over them, ensuring they are evenly coated.

4. Bake in the preheated oven for 25-30 minutes or until the chicken is cooked through and no longer pink in the center.

5. Remove from the oven and let the chicken rest for a few minutes before serving. Serve with your choice of steamed vegetables or a side salad.

Beef Stir-Fry with Broccoli and Bell Peppers

Ingredients:

- 1 pound beef sirloin, thinly sliced
- 2 tablespoons low-sodium soy sauce
- 1 tablespoon honey
- 1 tablespoon rice vinegar
- 2 cloves garlic, minced

- 1 teaspoon grated fresh ginger
- 2 tablespoons olive oil
- 2 cups broccoli florets
- 1 red bell pepper, sliced
- 1 yellow bell pepper, sliced
- Salt and pepper to taste

Instructions:

1. In a small bowl, whisk together the soy sauce, honey, rice vinegar, minced garlic, and grated ginger. Set aside.
2. Heat olive oil in a large skillet or wok over medium-high heat.
3. Add the sliced beef to the skillet and stir-fry for 3-4 minutes until browned. Remove the beef from the skillet and set aside.
4. In the same skillet, add the broccoli florets and sliced bell peppers. Stir-fry for 2-3 minutes until the vegetables are crisp-tender.
5. Return the beef to the skillet and pour the soy sauce mixture over the beef and vegetables. Stir-fry for an additional 2 minutes to coat everything evenly.

6. Season with salt and pepper to taste. Serve the beef stir-fry over steamed brown rice or quinoa.

Grilled Salmon with Dill Sauce

Ingredients:

- 4 salmon fillets
- 2 tablespoons olive oil
- 1 tablespoon fresh lemon juice
- 2 teaspoons dried dill
- Salt and pepper to taste

Dill Sauce:

- 1/2 cup Greek yogurt
- 1 tablespoon fresh lemon juice
- 1 tablespoon chopped fresh dill
- 1 teaspoon Dijon mustard
- Salt and pepper to taste

Instructions:

1. Preheat the grill to medium-high heat.
2. In a small bowl, whisk together the olive oil, lemon juice, dried dill, salt, and pepper.

3. Brush the salmon fillets with the olive oil mixture, coating both sides.

4. Place the salmon fillets on the preheated grill and cook for 4-5 minutes per side or until the fish flakes easily with a fork.

5. While the salmon is grilling, prepare the dill sauce. In another small bowl, combine the Greek yogurt, lemon juice, fresh dill, Dijon mustard, salt, and pepper. Mix well.

6. Remove the grilled salmon from the heat and serve with a dollop of dill sauce on top. Accompany with roasted sweet potatoes or a green salad.

Shrimp and Vegetable Stir-Fry

Ingredients:

- 1 pound large shrimp, peeled and deveined
- 2 tablespoons low-sodium soy sauce
- 1 tablespoon sesame oil
- 1 tablespoon honey
- 1 tablespoon rice vinegar
- 2 cloves garlic, minced
- 1 teaspoon grated fresh ginger

- 2 tablespoons olive oil

- 1 red bell pepper, sliced

- 1 yellow bell pepper, sliced

- 1 cup snap peas

- 1 small zucchini, sliced

- Salt and pepper to taste

- Optional: Sliced green onions for garnish

Instructions:

1. In a small bowl, whisk together the soy sauce, sesame oil, honey, rice vinegar, minced garlic, and grated ginger. Set aside.

2. Heat olive oil in a large skillet or wok over medium-high heat.

3. Add the shrimp to the skillet and stir-fry for 2-3 minutes until pink and cooked through. Remove the shrimp from the skillet and set aside.

4. In the same skillet, add the sliced bell peppers, snap peas, and sliced zucchini. Stir-fry for 2-3 minutes until the vegetables are crisp-tender.

5. Return the shrimp to the skillet and pour the soy sauce mixture over the shrimp and vegetables. Stir-

fry for an additional 2 minutes to coat everything evenly.

6. Season with salt and pepper to taste. Garnish with sliced green onions if desired. Serve the shrimp and vegetable stir-fry over steamed brown rice or quinoa.

Roasted Turkey Breast with Sweet Potatoes

Ingredients:

- 1 turkey breast (about 2 pounds)
- 2 tablespoons olive oil
- 1 teaspoon dried thyme
- 1 teaspoon dried rosemary
- 1 teaspoon paprika
- Salt and pepper to taste
- 2 medium sweet potatoes, peeled and cubed
- 1 red onion, sliced

Instructions:

1. Preheat the oven to 375°F (190°C).
2. Place the turkey breast in a roasting pan or baking dish.

3. In a small bowl, combine the olive oil, dried thyme, dried rosemary, paprika, salt, and pepper.

4. Rub the olive oil mixture all over the turkey breast, ensuring it is evenly coated.

5. Arrange the cubed sweet potatoes and sliced red onion around the turkey breast in the roasting pan.

6. Roast in the preheated oven for approximately 1 hour or until the turkey is cooked through and the sweet potatoes are tender.

7. Remove from the oven and let the turkey breast rest for a few minutes before slicing. Serve with roasted sweet potatoes and a side of steamed vegetables.

Quinoa Stuffed Bell Peppers

Ingredients:

- 4 bell peppers (any color), tops removed and seeds removed
- 1 cup cooked quinoa
- 1/2 pound ground turkey or lean ground beef
- 1/2 onion, diced
- 2 cloves garlic, minced
- 1/2 cup diced tomatoes

- 1/2 cup tomato sauce

- 1 teaspoon dried oregano

- 1 teaspoon dried basil

- Salt and pepper to taste

- Optional: Shredded mozzarella cheese for topping

Instructions:

1. Preheat the oven to 375°F (190°C).

2. In a large skillet, cook the ground turkey or lean

3. ground beef over medium heat until browned. Drain any excess fat.

4. Add the diced onion and minced garlic to the skillet and cook for 2-3 minutes until softened.

5. Stir in the cooked quinoa, diced tomatoes, tomato sauce, dried oregano, dried basil, salt, and pepper. Cook for an additional 2-3 minutes until heated through.

6. Stuff the bell peppers with the quinoa and meat mixture, packing it tightly.

7. Place the stuffed bell peppers in a baking dish and cover with foil. Bake in the preheated oven for 30 minutes.

8. Remove the foil and sprinkle shredded mozzarella cheese on top of each stuffed pepper if desired. Return to the oven and bake for an additional 5-10 minutes or until the cheese is melted and bubbly.

9. Remove from the oven and let the stuffed bell peppers cool slightly before serving.

Eggplant Parmesan

Ingredients:

- 1 large eggplant, sliced into rounds
- 2 eggs, beaten
- 1 cup breadcrumbs
- 1/2 cup grated Parmesan cheese
- 2 cups marinara sauce
- 1 cup shredded mozzarella cheese
- 1/4 cup chopped fresh basil
- Salt and pepper to taste
- Olive oil for frying

Instructions:

1. Preheat the oven to 375°F (190°C).

2. Dip each eggplant slice into the beaten eggs, then coat with breadcrumbs mixed with grated Parmesan cheese.

3. Heat olive oil in a large skillet over medium heat. Fry the coated eggplant slices for 2-3 minutes on each side until golden brown. Place the fried eggplant slices on a paper towel-lined plate to remove excess oil.

4. In a baking dish, spread a thin layer of marinara sauce. Arrange a layer of fried eggplant slices on top. Sprinkle with shredded mozzarella cheese, chopped fresh basil, salt, and pepper. Repeat the layers until all the eggplant slices are used, finishing with a layer of marinara sauce and shredded mozzarella cheese on top.

5. Cover the baking dish with foil and bake in the preheated oven for 20 minutes.

6. Remove the foil and continue baking for an additional 10-15 minutes or until the cheese is melted and bubbly.

7. Remove from the oven and let the eggplant Parmesan cool for a few minutes before serving. Garnish with additional chopped basil if desired.

Vegetable Curry with Brown Rice

Ingredients:

- 1 tablespoon olive oil
- 1 onion, diced
- 2 cloves garlic, minced
- 1 tablespoon curry powder
- 1 teaspoon ground cumin
- 1/2 teaspoon ground turmeric
- 1/2 teaspoon ground coriander
- 1/4 teaspoon cayenne pepper (optional, adjust to taste)
- 1 can (14 ounces) coconut milk
- 1 cup vegetable broth
- 2 carrots, sliced
- 1 zucchini, sliced
- 1 red bell pepper, sliced
- 1 cup cauliflower florets
- 1 cup frozen peas

- Salt and pepper to taste
- Cooked brown rice for serving

Instructions:

1. In a large skillet or pot, heat the olive oil over medium heat.
2. Add the diced onion and minced garlic to the skillet and cook for 2-3 minutes until softened.
3. Stir in the curry powder, ground cumin, ground turmeric, ground coriander, and cayenne pepper (if using). Cook for an additional minute until fragrant.
4. Pour in the coconut milk and vegetable broth. Stir well to combine.
5. Add the sliced carrots, zucchini, red bell pepper, cauliflower florets, and frozen peas to the skillet. Stir to coat the vegetables with the curry sauce.
6. Reduce the heat to low, cover, and simmer for 15-20 minutes or until the vegetables are tender.
7. Season with salt and pepper to taste. Serve the vegetable curry over cooked brown rice.

Mexican Cauliflower Rice Bowl

Ingredients:

- 1 head cauliflower, grated or processed into rice-like consistency
- 1 tablespoon olive oil
- 1/2 onion, diced
- 1 red bell pepper, diced
- 1 jalapeño, seeded and minced (optional)
- 2 cloves garlic, minced
- 1 teaspoon ground cumin
- 1 teaspoon chili powder
- 1 can (15 ounces) black beans, rinsed and drained
- 1 cup corn kernels
- 1/4 cup chopped fresh cilantro Juice of 1 lime
- Salt and pepper to taste
- Optional toppings: Sliced avocado, Greek yogurt, chopped tomatoes

Instructions:

1. Heat the olive oil in a large skillet over medium heat.
2. Add the diced onion, diced red bell pepper, minced jalapeño (if using), and minced garlic to the skillet.

Sauté for 2-3 minutes until the vegetables are softened.

3. Stir in the ground cumin and chili powder. Cook for an additional minute until fragrant.

4. Add the grated cauliflower to the skillet and stir to combine with the seasoned vegetables. Cook for 5-7 minutes until the cauliflower is tender.

5. Stir in the black beans, corn kernels, chopped fresh cilantro, lime juice, salt, and pepper. Cook for an additional 2-3 minutes to heat through.

6. Remove from heat and serve the Mexican cauliflower rice in bowls. Top with sliced avocado, a dollop of Greek yogurt, and chopped tomatoes if desired.

Baked Cod with Lemon and Herbs

Ingredients:

- 4 cod fillets
- 2 tablespoons olive oil
- 2 tablespoons fresh lemon juice
- 2 cloves garlic, minced
- 1 teaspoon dried dill

- 1 teaspoon dried parsley
- Salt and pepper to taste

Instructions:

1. Preheat the oven to 375°F (190°C).
2. Place the cod fillets in a baking dish.
3. In a small bowl, whisk together the olive oil, lemon juice, minced garlic, dried dill, dried parsley, salt, and pepper.
4. Pour the lemon and herb mixture over the cod fillets, ensuring they are evenly coated.
5. Bake in the preheated oven for 15-20 minutes or until the cod is opaque and flakes easily with a fork.
6. Remove from the oven and let the baked cod rest for a few minutes before serving. Serve with steamed vegetables or a side of quinoa.

Chapter 6: Snacks and Appetizers Recipes

In this Chapter of "The Acid Reflux Cookbook," you'll discover a variety of delightful and flavorful snacks and appetizers that are not only delicious but also gentle on your digestive system. These recipes are specially curated to help manage acid reflux symptoms while still satisfying your cravings. Let's dive into the delectable world of snacks and appetizers!

Roasted Red Pepper Hummus with Crudité

Ingredients:

- 1 can (15 ounces) chickpeas, drained and rinsed
- 2 roasted red peppers, peeled and seeded
- 3 tablespoons tahini
- 2 cloves garlic, minced
- 2 tablespoons fresh lemon juice
- 1 tablespoon olive oil
- 1/2 teaspoon ground cumin

- Salt and pepper to taste
- Crudité (such as carrot sticks, cucumber slices, and bell pepper strips), for serving

Instructions:

1. In a food processor, combine the chickpeas, roasted red peppers, tahini, minced garlic, lemon juice, olive oil, ground cumin, salt, and pepper.
2. Process the mixture until smooth and creamy, scraping down the sides as needed.
3. Transfer the hummus to a serving bowl and refrigerate for at least 30 minutes to allow the flavors to meld.
4. Serve the roasted red pepper hummus with an assortment of crudité for a refreshing and nutritious snack.

Guacamole with Baked Tortilla Chips

Ingredients:

- 2 ripe avocados
- 1/4 cup diced red onion

- 1 small tomato, diced
- 1 jalapeño pepper, seeded and minced
- 2 tablespoons fresh lime juice
- 2 tablespoons chopped fresh cilantro
- Salt and pepper to taste
- Baked tortilla chips, for serving

Instructions:

1. Cut the avocados in half, remove the pits, and scoop the flesh into a bowl.
2. Mash the avocados with a fork until desired consistency is reached (smooth or chunky).
3. Stir in the diced red onion, tomato, jalapeño pepper, lime juice, and chopped cilantro.
4. Season the guacamole with salt and pepper to taste.
5. Cover the bowl with plastic wrap, making sure it touches the surface of the guacamole to prevent browning, and refrigerate for 30 minutes.
6. Serve the guacamole with baked tortilla chips for a flavorful and satisfying snack.

Greek Yogurt and Fruit Dip

Ingredients:

- 1 cup Greek yogurt
- 2 tablespoons honey
- 1 teaspoon vanilla extract
- Assorted fresh fruits (such as strawberries, grapes, and pineapple), for dipping

Instructions:

1. In a small bowl, whisk together the Greek yogurt, honey, and vanilla extract until well combined.
2. Transfer the dip to a serving bowl and refrigerate for 15-20 minutes to allow the flavors to meld.
3. Arrange a variety of fresh fruits on a platter alongside the Greek yogurt dip.
4. Dip the fruits into the creamy and tangy Greek yogurt dip for a delightful and healthy snack.

Cucumber and Tomato Bruschetta

Ingredients:

- 1 English cucumber, diced
- 1 cup cherry tomatoes, halved

- 1/4 cup finely chopped red onion

- 2 tablespoons chopped fresh basil

- 1 tablespoon balsamic vinegar

- 1 tablespoon extra-virgin olive oil

- Salt and pepper to taste

- Sliced whole wheat baguette, toasted, for serving

Instructions:

1. In a bowl, combine the diced cucumber, cherry

2. tomatoes, red onion, chopped basil, balsamic vinegar, olive oil, salt, and pepper.

3. Toss the ingredients together until well coated.

4. Allow the cucumber and tomato mixture to sit at room temperature for 10-15 minutes to allow the flavors to meld.

5. Serve the cucumber and tomato bruschetta on toasted slices of whole wheat baguette for a refreshing and vibrant appetizer.

Baked Sweet Potato Fries

Ingredients:

- 2 large sweet potatoes, cut into thin strips

- 2 tablespoons olive oil
- 1 teaspoon paprika
- 1/2 teaspoon garlic powder
- 1/2 teaspoon onion powder
- 1/2 teaspoon dried thyme
- Salt and pepper to taste

Instructions:

1. Preheat the oven to 425°F (220°C) and line a baking sheet with parchment paper.
2. In a large bowl, toss the sweet potato strips with olive oil, paprika, garlic powder, onion powder, dried thyme, salt, and pepper until well coated.
3. Spread the sweet potato strips in a single layer on the prepared baking sheet.
4. Bake for 20-25 minutes, flipping the fries halfway through, until they are golden and crispy.
5. Remove from the oven and let them cool for a few minutes before serving.
6. Enjoy the guilt-free pleasure of crispy baked sweet potato fries as a flavorful and nutritious snack.

Oven-Baked Zucchini Chips

Ingredients:

- 2 medium zucchini, sliced into thin rounds
- 2 tablespoons olive oil
- 1/4 cup grated Parmesan cheese
- 1/2 teaspoon dried oregano
- 1/2 teaspoon garlic powder
- Salt and pepper to taste

Instructions:

1. Preheat the oven to 425°F (220°C) and line a baking sheet with parchment paper.
2. In a bowl, toss the zucchini slices with olive oil, grated Parmesan cheese, dried oregano, garlic powder, salt, and pepper until well coated.
3. Arrange the zucchini slices in a single layer on the prepared baking sheet.
4. Bake for 15-20 minutes, flipping the chips halfway through, until they are golden and crispy.
5. Allow the zucchini chips to cool slightly before serving.

6. Indulge in the savory and crunchy delight of oven-baked zucchini chips as a wholesome and flavorful snack.

Stuffed Mushrooms with Spinach and Feta

Ingredients:

- 16 large cremini mushrooms, stems removed
- 2 cups fresh spinach, chopped
- 1/4 cup crumbled feta cheese
- 2 cloves garlic, minced
- 1 tablespoon olive oil
- Salt and pepper to taste

Instructions:

1. Preheat the oven to 375°F (190°C) and line a baking sheet with parchment paper.
2. In a skillet, heat the olive oil over medium heat. Add the minced garlic and sauté for 1-2 minutes until fragrant.
3. Add the chopped spinach to the skillet and cook until wilted, about 3-4 minutes.

4. Remove the skillet from the heat and stir in the crumbled feta cheese. Season with salt and pepper to taste.

5. Fill each mushroom cap with the spinach and feta mixture and place them on the prepared baking sheet.

6. Bake for 15-20 minutes until the mushrooms are tender and the filling is lightly browned.

7. Allow the stuffed mushrooms to cool for a few minutes before serving.

8. Delight in the savory combination of flavors in these stuffed mushrooms with spinach and feta as a delectable appetizer.

Quinoa and Black Bean Salad Cups

Ingredients:

- 1 cup cooked quinoa
- 1 cup black beans, rinsed and drained
- 1/2 cup diced bell peppers (assorted colors)
- 1/4 cup chopped fresh cilantro
- 2 tablespoons fresh lime juice
- 1 tablespoon extra-virgin olive oil
- 1/2 teaspoon ground cumin

- Salt and pepper to taste

- Lettuce leaves, for serving

Instructions:

1. In a bowl, combine the cooked quinoa, black beans, diced bell peppers, chopped cilantro, lime juice, olive oil, ground cumin, salt, and pepper. Toss until well mixed.

2. Refrigerate the quinoa and black bean mixture for 15-20 minutes to allow the flavors to meld.

3. Spoon the chilled quinoa and black bean salad into lettuce leaves, creating cups.

4. Serve these quinoa and black bean salad cups as a refreshing and protein-packed appetizer.

Smoked Salmon Roll-Ups

Ingredients:

- 4 whole wheat tortillas

- 4 ounces smoked salmon

- 4 tablespoons cream cheese

- 1/4 cup diced red onion

- 2 tablespoons chopped fresh dill

- Juice of 1/2 lemon
- Salt and pepper to taste

Instructions:

1. Lay the whole wheat tortillas flat on a clean surface.
2. Spread 1 tablespoon of cream cheese evenly on each tortilla.
3. Place smoked salmon slices on top of the cream cheese layer.
4. Sprinkle the diced red onion, chopped fresh dill, lemon juice, salt, and pepper over the salmon.
5. Roll up the tortillas tightly and slice them into bite-sized roll-ups.
6. Secure each roll-up with a toothpick if desired.
7. Serve the smoked salmon roll-ups as elegant and flavorful appetizers.

Spicy Edamame

Ingredients:

- 2 cups frozen edamame, thawed
- 1 tablespoon soy sauce
- 1 tablespoon sriracha sauce

- 1 teaspoon sesame oil

- 1 teaspoon sesame seeds (optional)

Instructions:

1. Steam or boil the thawed edamame until tender, following the package instructions.
2. Drain the edamame and transfer them to a bowl.
3. In a separate small bowl, whisk together the soy sauce, sriracha sauce, and sesame oil.
4. Pour the sauce over the edamame and toss until well coated.
5. Sprinkle sesame seeds on top for an extra touch of flavor and presentation (optional).
6. Serve the spicy edamame as a zesty and protein-rich snack.

Chapter 7: Dessert Recipes

In this chapter, we will explore a variety of delicious dessert recipes that are not only satisfying to the sweet tooth but also suitable for individuals managing acid reflux. These desserts focus on using ingredients that are gentle on the digestive system while still providing plenty of flavor and indulgence. From fruity delights to creamy treats, get ready to enjoy these mouthwatering desserts without worrying about triggering acid reflux symptoms.

Berry Chia Pudding

Ingredients:

- 1 cup almond milk
- 3 tablespoons chia seeds
- 1 tablespoon maple syrup or honey
- 1/2 teaspoon vanilla extract
- 1/2 cup mixed berries (strawberries, blueberries, raspberries)

Instructions:

1. In a bowl, combine the almond milk, chia seeds, maple syrup (or honey), and vanilla extract. Stir well to ensure the chia seeds are evenly distributed.

2. Let the mixture sit for 10 minutes, stirring occasionally to prevent clumping.

3. Cover the bowl and refrigerate overnight or for at least 4 hours to allow the chia seeds to absorb the liquid and thicken.

4. When ready to serve, give the chia pudding a good stir to break up any clumps.

5. Layer the chia pudding and mixed berries in a glass or bowl, alternating between the two.

6. Top with an extra sprinkle of chia seeds or additional berries, if desired.

7. Enjoy this refreshing and nutritious berry chia pudding as a guilt-free dessert or even as a healthy breakfast option.

Baked Apples with Cinnamon and Almonds

Ingredients:

- 2 medium-sized apples (Granny Smith or your preferred variety)
- 2 tablespoons chopped almonds
- 1 tablespoon honey
- 1 teaspoon ground cinnamon
- 1/2 teaspoon coconut oil

Instructions:

1. Preheat the oven to 350°F (175°C).
2. Core the apples using an apple corer or a knife, leaving the bottom intact. This will create a well in the center for the filling.
3. In a small bowl, combine the chopped almonds, honey, cinnamon, and coconut oil. Mix well.
4. Stuff the almond mixture into the well of each apple, distributing it evenly between the two.
5. Place the stuffed apples on a baking sheet or in a baking dish.
6. Bake in the preheated oven for approximately 25-30 minutes or until the apples are tender and the filling is golden brown.

7. Remove from the oven and let them cool slightly before serving.

8. These baked apples with cinnamon and almonds make a delightful dessert on their own or can be enjoyed with a dollop of Greek yogurt or a sprinkle of granola for added texture.

Coconut Yogurt Parfait with Mixed Berries

Ingredients:

- 1 cup coconut yogurt (dairy-free option)
- 1/2 cup mixed berries (strawberries, blueberries, raspberries)
- 2 tablespoons shredded coconut
- 2 tablespoons chopped almonds or walnuts
- 1 tablespoon honey or maple syrup (optional)

Instructions:

1. In a glass or a bowl, layer the coconut yogurt, mixed berries, shredded coconut, and chopped nuts.

2. Repeat the layers until all the ingredients are used, finishing with a sprinkle of berries and a small handful of shredded coconut on top.

3. Drizzle with honey or maple syrup, if desired, for a touch of sweetness.

4. Serve this refreshing and creamy coconut yogurt parfait as a delightful dessert or even as a healthy snack option.

Chocolate Avocado Mousse

Ingredients:

- 2 ripe avocados
- 1/4 cup cocoa powder (unsweetened)
- 1/4 cup maple syrup or honey
- 1/4 cup almond milk
- 1 teaspoon vanilla extract
- Pinch of sea salt
- Fresh berries or chopped nuts for garnish (optional)

Instructions:

1. Scoop the flesh of the avocados into a blender or food processor.

2. Add the cocoa powder, maple syrup (or honey),
   almond milk, vanilla extract, and a pinch of sea salt.

3. Blend until smooth and creamy, scraping down the
   sides as needed to ensure everything is well
   incorporated.

4. Transfer the chocolate avocado mousse to individual
   serving bowls or glasses.

5. Refrigerate for at least 1 hour to allow the mousse to
   set and the flavors to meld.

6. Before serving, garnish with fresh berries or chopped
   nuts, if desired, to add a pop of color and texture.

7. Indulge in this rich and velvety chocolate avocado
   mousse, a dessert that combines decadence with the
   health benefits of avocados.

Almond Flour Banana Bread

Ingredients:

- 2 ripe bananas, mashed
- 3 large eggs
- 1/4 cup coconut oil, melted
- 1/4 cup honey or maple syrup
- 1 teaspoon vanilla extract

- 2 cups almond flour
- 1 teaspoon baking powder
- 1/2 teaspoon baking soda
- 1/2 teaspoon ground cinnamon
- Pinch of salt

Instructions:

1. Preheat the oven to 350°F (175°C). Grease a loaf pan with coconut oil or line it with parchment paper.
2. In a large bowl, combine the mashed bananas, eggs, melted coconut oil, honey (or maple syrup), and vanilla extract. Mix well.
3. In a separate bowl, whisk together the almond flour, baking powder, baking soda, ground cinnamon, and salt.
4. Gradually add the dry ingredients to the wet ingredients, stirring until just combined. Be careful not to overmix.
5. Pour the batter into the prepared loaf pan, spreading it evenly.
6. Bake in the preheated oven for 40-45 minutes or until a toothpick inserted into the center comes out clean.

7. Remove the banana bread from the oven and let it cool in the pan for 10 minutes.

8. Transfer the bread to a wire rack to cool completely before slicing.

9. Enjoy a slice of this moist and flavorful almond flour banana bread, perfect for a sweet treat or a breakfast on the go.

Mango Sorbet

Ingredients:

- 2 ripe mangoes, peeled and pitted
- 1 tablespoon fresh lime juice
- 1 tablespoon honey or maple syrup (optional)

Instructions:

1. Cut the mango flesh into chunks and place them in a blender or food processor.

2. Add the fresh lime juice and honey (or maple syrup), if using.

3. Blend until smooth and creamy, pausing to scrape down the sides if necessary.

4. Taste the mixture and adjust the sweetness by adding more honey or maple syrup if desired.

5. Pour the mango mixture into a shallow dish or a loaf pan.

6. Cover with plastic wrap and freeze for at least 4 hours or until firm.

7. When ready to serve, let the sorbet sit at room temperature for a few minutes to soften slightly.

8. Scoop the mango sorbet into bowls or cones, and enjoy this refreshing and tropical dessert that's bursting with mango goodness.

Grilled Pineapple with Honey and Mint

Ingredients:

- 1 pineapple, peeled, cored, and cut into rings or wedges
- 2 tablespoons honey
- Fresh mint leaves, chopped

Instructions:

1. Preheat the grill to medium heat.

2. Brush the pineapple rings or wedges with honey, ensuring they are evenly coated.

3. Place the pineapple pieces on the grill and cook for 2-3 minutes per side, or until grill marks appear and the pineapple caramelizes slightly.

4. Remove the grilled pineapple from the heat and let it cool for a minute.

5. Sprinkle with freshly chopped mint leaves for a burst of freshness and aroma.

6. Serve the grilled pineapple as a delightful dessert on its own or alongside a scoop of vanilla yogurt or a sprinkle of toasted coconut flakes.

Roasted Peaches with Greek Yogurt

Ingredients:

- 2 ripe peaches, halved and pitted
- 1 tablespoon coconut oil, melted
- 1 tablespoon honey or maple syrup
- 1/2 teaspoon ground cinnamon
- Greek yogurt for serving
- Chopped almonds or walnuts for garnish (optional)

Instructions:

1. Preheat the oven to 375°F (190°C).
2. In a small bowl, combine the melted coconut oil, honey (or maple syrup), and ground cinnamon.
3. Place the peach halves on a baking sheet or in a baking dish, cut side up.
4. Brush the peach halves with the coconut oil mixture, making sure they are well coated.
5. Roast in the preheated oven for 15-20 minutes or until the peaches are tender and caramelized.
6. Remove from the oven and let them cool slightly.
7. Serve each roasted peach half with a dollop of Greek yogurt and a sprinkle of chopped almonds or walnuts, if desired.
8. Savor the natural sweetness of the roasted peaches combined with the creaminess of Greek yogurt in this simple yet delightful dessert.

Strawberry Almond Crumble

Ingredients:

- 2 cups fresh strawberries, hulled and sliced
- 1 tablespoon lemon juice

- 1/4 cup almond flour
- 1/4 cup rolled oats
- 2 tablespoons chopped almonds
- 2 tablespoons honey or maple syrup
- 1 tablespoon coconut oil, melted
- 1/2 teaspoon ground cinnamon
- Pinch of salt

Instructions:

1. Preheat the oven to 375°F (190°C).
2. In a bowl, combine the sliced strawberries and lemon juice. Toss gently to coat the strawberries and set aside.
3. In a separate bowl, combine the almond flour, rolled oats, chopped almonds, honey (or maple syrup), melted coconut oil, ground cinnamon, and a pinch of salt. Mix well to form a crumbly texture.
4. Place the strawberry mixture in a baking dish or individual ramekins.
5. Sprinkle the almond crumble mixture evenly over the strawberries.

6. Bake in the preheated oven for 20-25 minutes or until the strawberries are bubbly and the crumble topping is golden brown.

7. Remove from the oven and let it cool slightly before serving.

8. Enjoy the delightful combination of sweet strawberries and crunchy almond crumble in this comforting dessert.

Blueberry Coconut Ice Cream

Ingredients:

- 2 cans full-fat coconut milk
- 1 cup frozen blueberries
- 1/4 cup honey or maple syrup
- 1 teaspoon vanilla extract

Instructions:

1. In a blender or food processor, combine the coconut milk, frozen blueberries, honey (or maple syrup), and vanilla extract.

2. Blend until smooth and creamy, ensuring that the blueberries are fully incorporated.

3. Pour the mixture into an ice cream maker and churn according to the manufacturer's instructions.

4. Transfer the churned ice cream to a lidded container and freeze for at least 2 hours or until firm.

5. When ready to serve, let the ice cream sit at room temperature for a few minutes to soften.

6. Scoop the blueberry coconut ice cream into bowls or cones, and enjoy this luscious and dairy-free treat bursting with blueberry flavor.

Chapter 8: Smoothie Recipes

Smoothies are not only delicious and refreshing but can also be a fantastic way to incorporate nutritious ingredients into your diet. In this chapter, we will explore ten delightful smoothie recipes that are not only satisfying to the taste buds but also provide a host of health benefits. So, grab your blender and let's dive into the world of revitalizing smoothies!

Green Detox Smoothie

Ingredients:

- 1 cup fresh spinach leaves
- 1 green apple, cored and chopped
- 1 ripe banana
- 1 small cucumber, peeled and chopped
- ½ lemon, juiced
- ½ cup coconut water
- Ice cubes (optional)

Instructions:

1. Place all the ingredients into a blender.

2. Blend until smooth and creamy.

3. If desired, add ice cubes for a chilled texture.

4. Pour into a glass and enjoy this detoxifying green elixir.

Banana Berry Smoothie

Ingredients:

- 1 ripe banana
- 1 cup mixed berries (such as strawberries, blueberries, and raspberries)
- 1 cup unsweetened almond milk
- 1 tablespoon honey or maple syrup (optional)
- Ice cubes (optional)

Instructions:

1. Add the banana, mixed berries, almond milk, and sweetener (if using) to the blender.

2. Blend until all the ingredients are well combined.

3. For a colder smoothie, include a handful of ice cubes and blend again.

4. Pour into a glass and savor the fruity goodness of this delightful smoothie.

Tropical Turmeric Smoothie

Ingredients:

- 1 cup frozen mango chunks
- ½ ripe banana
- ½ cup pineapple chunks
- 1 teaspoon turmeric powder
- 1 cup coconut milk
- 1 tablespoon chia seeds (optional)

Instructions:

1. Place the frozen mango chunks, banana, pineapple chunks, turmeric powder, coconut milk, and chia seeds (if using) into the blender.
2. Blend until the mixture becomes smooth and creamy.
3. Pour into a glass and transport yourself to a tropical paradise with each sip of this vibrant smoothie.

Spinach and Pineapple Smoothie

Ingredients:

- 2 cups fresh spinach leaves
- 1 cup frozen pineapple chunks
- 1 ripe banana
- 1 cup coconut water
- 1 tablespoon flaxseeds (optional)

Instructions:

1. Combine the spinach leaves, frozen pineapple chunks, ripe banana, coconut water, and flaxseeds (if using) in the blender.
2. Blend until all the ingredients are thoroughly mixed and the smoothie reaches your desired consistency.
3. Pour into a glass and enjoy the perfect blend of sweetness and freshness in this green delight.

Mango Ginger Smoothie

Ingredients:

- 1 ½ cups frozen mango chunks
- 1 tablespoon fresh ginger, grated
- ½ cup Greek yogurt
- 1 cup unsweetened almond milk
- 1 tablespoon honey or maple syrup (optional)

- Ice cubes (optional)

Instructions:

1. Add the frozen mango chunks, grated ginger, Greek yogurt, almond milk, and sweetener (if using) to the blender.
2. Blend until the mixture turns smooth and creamy.
3. If desired, include a few ice cubes for a frostier texture.
4. Pour into a glass and revel in the tropical fusion of mango and ginger flavors.

Blueberry Avocado Smoothie

Ingredients:

- 1 cup fresh or frozen blueberries
- ½ ripe avocado
- 1 cup spinach leaves
- 1 tablespoon almond butter
- 1 cup almond milk
- 1 tablespoon honey or maple syrup (optional)

Instructions:

1. Combine the blueberries, avocado, spinach leaves, almond butter, almond milk, and sweetener (if using) in the blender.

2. Blend until all the ingredients are well incorporated and the smoothie becomes velvety.

3. Pour into a glass and indulge in the creamy texture and antioxidant-rich flavors of this delightful smoothie.

Raspberry Beet Smoothie

Ingredients:

- 1 cup fresh or frozen raspberries
- 1 small cooked beet, peeled and chopped
- ½ cup Greek yogurt
- 1 tablespoon honey or maple syrup (optional)
- 1 cup almond milk
- Ice cubes (optional)

Instructions:

1. Add the raspberries, cooked beet, Greek yogurt, sweetener (if using), almond milk, and ice cubes (if desired) to the blender.

2. Blend until all the ingredients are thoroughly mixed and the smoothie turns vibrant pink.

3. Pour into a glass and relish the unique combination of sweet raspberries and earthy beets in this nutritious smoothie.

Kiwi Kale Smoothie

Ingredients:

- 2 ripe kiwis, peeled and sliced
- 1 cup kale leaves
- 1 ripe banana
- 1 cup coconut water
- 1 tablespoon lime juice
- Ice cubes (optional)

Instructions:

1. Place the kiwis, kale leaves, ripe banana, coconut water, lime juice, and ice cubes (if using) into the blender.

2. Blend until all the ingredients are well blended and the smoothie achieves a smooth consistency.

3. Pour into a glass and enjoy the invigorating flavors of kiwi and kale in this energizing smoothie.

Papaya Passion Smoothie

Ingredients:

- 1 cup ripe papaya, peeled and seeded
- 1 passion fruit, pulp scooped out
- ½ cup Greek yogurt
- 1 cup coconut water
- 1 tablespoon honey or maple syrup (optional)

Instructions:

1. Add the papaya, passion fruit pulp, Greek yogurt, coconut water, and sweetener (if using) to the blender.
2. Blend until all the ingredients are thoroughly combined and the smoothie becomes velvety.
3. Pour into a glass and revel in the tropical tanginess of this papaya and passion fruit blend.

Almond Butter and Chocolate Smoothie

Ingredients:

- 2 tablespoons almond butter
- 1 ripe banana
- 1 tablespoon cocoa powder
- 1 cup almond milk
- 1 tablespoon honey or maple syrup (optional)
- Ice cubes (optional)

Instructions:

1. Combine the almond butter, ripe banana, cocoa powder, almond milk, and sweetener (if using) in the blender.
2. Blend until the ingredients are well mixed and the smoothie turns creamy.
3. For a colder and thicker texture, include a handful of ice cubes and blend again.
4. Pour into a glass and relish the indulgent flavors of almond butter and chocolate in this delightful smoothie.

CONCLUSION

In the final chapter of "The Acid Reflux Cookbook," we come to a point of reflection and consolidation. Think back to when you first started this cookbook. Remember the initial challenges you faced and the uncertainties that lingered in your mind. Perhaps you were overwhelmed by the idea of giving up certain foods or concerned about finding suitable alternatives. But as you immersed yourself in the pages of this cookbook, you gained confidence, learned new cooking techniques, and discovered flavorful ingredients that can be enjoyed without triggering acid reflux symptoms.

Consider the positive changes you have experienced along the way. Have you noticed a reduction in acid reflux episodes? Do you feel more energized and less burdened by discomfort? Take note of these improvements and celebrate your achievements, no matter how small they may seem. Recognizing your progress will reinforce your commitment to maintaining a healthy lifestyle.

Maintaining a Healthy Lifestyle Beyond the Cookbook

While this cookbook has provided you with a wealth of information and mouthwatering recipes, it's essential to remember that it is just one piece of the puzzle. The acid reflux diet is a long-term commitment to your well-being, and it goes beyond the confines of this book. As you move forward, keep the following principles in mind to maintain a healthy lifestyle and manage acid reflux effectively:

1. Stay Consistent: The success of the acid reflux diet lies in its consistency. Try to adhere to the guidelines outlined in this cookbook on a regular basis. Consistency will help minimize acid reflux symptoms and promote overall digestive health.

2. Listen to Your Body: Each person's experience with acid reflux is unique. Pay attention to how your body reacts to different foods and lifestyle choices. Make adjustments accordingly to find what works best for you.

3. Keep a Food Journal: Maintaining a food journal can be a valuable tool in understanding your triggers and identifying patterns. Record what you eat, when you eat it, and any symptoms that arise. This information

will help you make informed decisions about your diet.

4. Seek Professional Advice: While this cookbook provides general information and guidance, consulting with a healthcare professional or registered dietitian is always recommended. They can offer personalized advice based on your specific needs and medical history.

5. Prioritize Stress Management: Stress can exacerbate acid reflux symptoms. Incorporate stress management techniques into your daily routine, such as meditation, yoga, deep breathing exercises, or engaging in activities that bring you joy.

Final Thoughts and Encouragement

Completing "The Acid Reflux Cookbook" is just the beginning of your acid reflux journey. By implementing the knowledge and skills you have gained, you are equipped to make lasting changes that will positively impact your health and well-being. Remember, progress takes time, and setbacks may occur, but do not be discouraged. Each day presents an opportunity to make choices that align with your goal of managing acid reflux and living a vibrant life.